One Way Ticket to Slimming

ALEX SUMA

ISBN-13: 978-1494252519
ISBN-10: 1494252511

DEDICATION

This book is for everyone! Not only for the people who want to lose weight subjected to frustrating diets. Not only for those who after all the effort again returned weight. This book is for anyone who wants to achieve top body form in his life, in a mental and physical level! This book is for anyone who loves and appreciates himself!

CONTENTS

ACKNOWLEDGMENTS

I love to write exciting stories, stories about people and events that change the human senses, but instead, I wrote this book. I, like many others, had long battle with my body and weight. After trying everything, I found my own way for losing weight. I have successfully managed hundreds of people to lose their weight with my methods. They are the one who convinced me to write this ebook.

ONE WAY TICKET TO SLIMMING

You have problems with you weight? You have been in constant battle with your extra kilograms? You slim and then gain weight back again and sometimes even double the kilos lost? You have tried all popular diets and you are still away from the shape you wish for? You have despaired and given it up? But I am telling you not to! I know why you are losing these battles! There are some little things you have to change in order to succeed! There are some facts that you need to know! It is even possible that you know these things but I will make u understand them. This is the missing link in all diets that you have tried by now. That is why you have not succeeded yet!

I know that you are fed up with being fat or plump. I will tell you what to do about it and if you really understand what I have to say I guarantee that you will get slim no matter if you are sixteen or sixty.

I am not disputing any of the diets or dietary regimes but I'll immediately say that I am not a supporter of starving for the purpose of slimming.

I haven't discovered the warm water and I know you haven't either. I know you have read a lot on the topic and you know almost everything about the good and the bad carbohydrates, about the foods that lead to slimming and about the food supplements that possess magical slimming properties. Very often though people who can't lose the surplus weight are not weak but not well informed enough. May be the next pages hide the secret that has been stopping you from slimming until now. I won't let you to go on starving and I won't deprive you of anything. This book is not the next revolutionary diet but about the facts of nutrition and about a healthy life style. You will understand why do you put on weight and can't lose it! And you will learn what to do in order to get and stay slim permanently!

You have to know that if you feel sleepy or lazy or you forget anything in minutes – the true perpetrator is the food you eat.

"You are what you eat" – the ancient Indian medicine is trumpeting for centuries and this now has found its scientific support and explanation.

New research has proved that if someone has been eating too much fatty products for more than ten days he or she may get to feel too lazy because of that.

Cambridge scientists have experimented with two groups of rats.

The first group of rata was on a diet – they were given low fat foods. The other rats were having food rich in calories and in quantities - as much as they wanted.

The two groups had to pass a complex labyrinth. The slim rats that have had healthy food passed it easy and quickly without making a single mistake.

Their rivals though felt lost and going in circles. In addition it was found that their muscles were receiving less oxygen for the period of the rich food nourishing.

The experts investigated the reasons for that problem on a cellular level and especially in the mitochondria of the muscle cells. The results showed increased levels of protein and that was causing them being less effective.

Getting fat, diabetes and the heart diseases very often are due to having too many foods too rich in fats.

And because of the quick pace of our everyday life we often do not pay enough attention to what we eat.

But we really should!

Why am I not able to lose weight? Why am I always hungry and fat? I lost a lot of kilos and then gained them back but three times heavier! There is not a single diet I haven't tried! And I know these are exactly the questions you have in mind too, don't you?

Here – I will answer your questions! WHY CAN'T YOU LOOSE WEIGHT? I WILL ALSO TELL YOU HOW TO DO IT!

Please stop with statements of the sort: "I don't eat anything and I am still getting fat", "there is some disorder in my metabolism that's why I am getting fat", "I'll put on weight even if I have a glass of water"! You are just kidding me! No one puts weight out of water and your metabolism is not at its best because of the bad food u eat! And you do not pull my leg saying that you do not eat anything!

I forgot – we would better speak informally as you are there with my book and in a way it is like being there with me. It is like we are having a nice talk. We shall break the ice faster that way.

If you listen to me and not be lazy I promise that this battle with the overweight will be your last. You will never be fat again. But most important is that I will not let you stay hungry neither shall I deprive you of the foods that you adore.

YOU SHOULD KNOW THAT:

1. using only a diet – you will burn fats but also muscles;
2. diet plus exercises – that burns fats;
3. only exercises – that does not lead to losing weight.

If you fall to the group of people who hate physical exercising now you are a bit disappointed! I am comforting you now that you can go without gymnastics. I will explain later though why I recommend that you have some physical training. Then you will have to decide for yourself and chose what to do. You are an adult and you know that there is no complete happiness!

And now as we know that fat people like to eat we shall start with some good news. When can you eat the things you love?

.

A FEAST SHOULD BE A FEAST! NO RESTRICTIONS!

On the celebration night everything should be perfect! So no diets when we celebrate! I am the best, aren't I?

But there hardly can be more than two celebrations a month except for December when there are much more.

If you are on a diet:

You can have a light breakfast on the celebration days. After that you should better stay hungry all day – meaning you can have just water, tea without sugar, no fruit juices either.

Then on the celebration night you indulge yourself as much as you want. But let it be going in stages.

Festivities have started – at the beginning you can go around and try everything on the table. Then I recommend a ten minutes rest. If you are still hungry you can make a second round – everything that is there is permitted to you. Have another ten minutes rest or more. Then maybe you will have a third round. At this point you should be quite full because on celebration tables there are usually more 7-8-9 meals and you haven't actually been in much effort "running" around that table.

If you want to keep your shape

At times of celebrations you do not have to feel troubled. Be comfortable, behave as a happy person and do not give much thinking on what is healthy and what is heavy at the table of the feast. The only thing you have to observe here is to eat as much as you want at only one meal for the day. Do not get very full at breakfast, lunch and dinner. You cannot feel well that way; your energy will be low if you constantly have food that needs to be processed in your stomach.

On the contrary – if you can wait with the food you will feel motivated and be looking forward to the feast and the pleasure of getting full. You will have a day of nice expectations with the tasty things prepared for you there and your spirit will be high at the celebration. You will not feel heavy and swollen and too full. You will be light, happy and pleasantly impatient.

HOW TO MEASURE YOUR WEIGHT DURING AND AFTER FEATS?

When your body is receiving more food and especially carbohydrates this leads to retaining more liquids in the tissues. First your stomach will have a larger load in (I know that one can get about one kilo of food in one go) and second – your tissues will keep about a kilo of liquids more than usual. So the scales will show two kilos more. Even more then that! This is due to the fact that some people can down more than one kilo of food and respectively - retain more than a kilo of liquids. They will see that they have gained more than two kilos just for one rich dinner.

Does it mean that you have gained two kilos of fats? No, it does not. Nothing dramatic has happened and you have not put on weight; you can stay calm.

To retain less water you have to drink more water. This will also help you to get back to your previous weight. The more water you drink, the faster you are freeing your body of the liquids retained – and so you solve that problem. It usually takes about three days of keeping your diet or lifestyle to get back to your previous weight.

Attention!

Weight is a very inaccurate measure. Scales can go back and forth by two or more kilos due to food in the stomach and water retained in the soft tissues. But it doesn't mean that you have become fatter by two kilos. You would better get to measure the circumference of the waist, hips and thighs. That is much better index of your results.

BUT

PLEASE NOTE THAT I SPEAK ABOUT SURFAIT ONCE A DAY. AND I DON'T MEAN DO IT REGULARLY.

Alternative nutrition

We can often hear and read about eating small portions five-six times a day. I also believed in that at the beginning. There are periods in which this might be all right. If for example you start a regime for lowering the fats in your food then your portions are getting poorer and that leads to discomfort and hunger until getting used to the new daily calories. Then having small portions but regularly helps you to stop the ravenous hunger and excessive eating is prevented. But the content by the satisfaction of your huger is missing. There is a transitional period of about two, three or four months during which eating 5 times a day is good and helps to reduce the quantity of food you have become used to and in the same time keeps levels of blood sugar stable.

Long term, though, I think it is better to go to eating two or three times a day. This is good for several reasons.

Social reasons

You can have a light breakfast and after that you can spend the whole working day on water and tea (without sugar or honey). In the evenings people (family, friends) usually get together to get relaxed, loose the stress and feel content and happiness – by the company, conversations, emotions that we share and of course – by the food (meaning substantial eating). Eating is a need but also it is a pleasure. The content that we feel when we satisfy our hunger is needed and awaited for most of us.

If you eat two times a day you can eat whatever you want because you cannot have too much food and if occasionally you do that food will not be entirely assimilated. Nevertheless I recommend that you should get full with quality foods and not with flour and sugar but the choice remains yours because we people are different. You can even eat three times a day but between the meals you must not eat anything, not even a salty sticklette;

you may have water and tea without sugar or honey. You have to get used to eating only at the times you really sit down to eat. Do not eat or nibble anything between meals!

Health reason

Lately many people develop insulin resistance. This is a pre-diabetic condition where the insulin cannot get the sugars of the blood into the cells and the result is high levels of sugar in the blood and additional quantities of insulin produced by the pancreas. That exhausts it until it is not able to produce enough insulin or even stops – that is diabetes – no insulin. That is why I think that eating very often is not good for the health – besides everything else it increases the sugar in the blood too often.

We do not know the reasons that lead to insulin resistance and diabetes. I have this idea that is based on the evolution and a bit of sixth sense if you please – meaning I haven't got proof. I think, though, that eating too often, the easy access to food and the lack of physical activities lead to insulin resistance.

I think that if we provoke insulin production not so often that should make us more sensitive to it. And that means to eat food in bigger periods because eating leads to insulin secretion.

Evolutionary reason

Having in mind evolution – people did not have refrigerators or grocery shops to buy food whenever they want. Getting food used to involve looking for it - physical activity at conditions of hunger – for it used to be going when food supply is over. That mean eating could not have been a regular process occurring in every three or four hours. People used to eat much when food is plenty and then have a period of hunger when the food supply is over – it means relatively irregular periods of hunger and surfeit.

In conclusion

If you clear you're eating habits of flour (all cereals) and sugar, you can eat whatever you want and as much as you want.

You eat fast and sound and then you wait until you get hungry again. You will see that it will take you about six or eight hours to get hungry again. Then you sit to have your meal and you will find out that the day is over.

Here are some foods that you better eventually stop (in a period of one or two years) or you may have them rarely enough – bread, bakeries, cakes, cookies, pretzels, crackers, biscuits, pizzas, pasta, salty sticks and the like.

The foods that supply you with sugar – you would better substitute them by fruit.

4 ENOUGH OF THE CELEBRATION DINNERS

Fests are over and with them we are through with going around the luxury dinner table as well as with compromises.

Before we go on would like to specify what a diet means. Diet sounds scary! Sounds like being destitute, uncomfortable and grim. May be you would prefer that I used another word.

So what diet is and what it is not.

Diet is to control what you get to eat and drink aiming at definite results – regarding health, beauty, sport or religion. Results can be measured by kilograms, muscle mass, fats, and so on. But of course you know that.

In other words diet is a nutrition regime following certain rules and depending on the aims that are defined in advance. Diets are basically several   types:

- slimming diet;
- diet to support the condition of the body;
- diet to achieve and sustain certain sport results;
- diet to put on weight;
- professional diets aiming at the specific requirements of a certain job.
- religious diets – fasts;
- diets to heal different diseases;

So next time you hear some one saying that he or she is on diet – you may ask what is the goal of that diet. Have in mind that sports people, body builders, gymnasts – they all preserve strict nutrition regimes and hard diets according to the requirements of their sport.

First and most important thing that we have to begin with – that is motivation. You have to be motivated! Define a goal for yourself – how mush kilograms do you want to loose! Visualize your goal, buy the clothes of the size you aim at and imagine yourself in them – one day you will really put them on – of course. You set your mind aiming at this success and get to believe in it. I presume you have read "Mind Power" by John Kehoe as well as the "Secret". If not – then you have to.

There is an original thought too: "Sow a thought and you reap an action; sow an act and you reap a habit; sow a habit and you reap a character; sow a character and you reap a destiny." Ralph Waldo Emerson

Then you through away your scales and buy a tape measure!

You see friends who you haven't seen for a long time. "Wow, you look wonderful, you have slimmed so much!" Do they know how many kilos have you lost? No, they don't but they _can see_ you – your waist is slimmer, bottom is smaller, thighs are elegant. They can see your _circumferences_. They have no idea how much do you weigh.

You wake up and go to the scales and – nightmare – you weigh 1.50 kilos more then yesterday. So you have become fatter! Your world is all in ruins. You keep the regime, do the exercises and at the end you are putting on weight. At least you could have had some nice eating – then you will know what exactly caused your fatting. Then, when you put on your trousers you miss to notice that they are not tight for you. You have to make up your mind of today - you will not eat and you will exercise hard or you will eat as much as you want – because your efforts are fruitless all the same. And you cannot decide – the scales have confused you so much.

When does the scale lie?

11

For those women who want to just get their body firmer the scales are useless because while they are training they build muscles and so they weigh heavier. At the same time they reduce the fats of the body and the result is that no change of weight occurs. It says the same. It is even possible that the circumferences of the body become visibly smaller and the person is obviously slimmer but the kilos get higher. That is due to the physical training and muscle building. And there is no way to be physically active and not build some muscles.

If you want to make your body slimmer and firmer you don't have to watch the scales but the measures of the body. Write down the measures you have before getting to a regime – waist, hips, and thighs – left and right, leg calves – left and right, arm – the biceps at rest. If you have a well visible waist – get the smallest circumference. There are people whose waist is hardly the smallest circumference – the men with beer bellies and bigger women. Hips, thighs, leg calves and arms – take measures several times and put down the smallest circumference. The idea is that from that moment on they have to become smaller and smaller. That's why you will take the biggest circumference and watch its changing. Also – you do not need to take the measures at one and the same place every time – taking the measures is quite subjective and not a stable parameter. You can monitor just one of the thighs – if the left is slimming, the right is also slimming for sure. It's just normal that there is a certain difference between the circumferences of the left and right thigh.

If you want to make your body slimmer and firmer you don't have to watch the scales but the measures of the body. Write down the measures you have before getting to a regime – waist, hips, and thighs – left and right, leg calves – left and right, arm – the biceps at rest. If you have a well visible waist – get the smallest circumference. There are people whose waist is hardly the smallest circumference – the men with beer bellies and bigger women. Hips, thighs, leg calves and arms – take measures several times and put down the smallest circumference. The idea is that from that moment on they have to become smaller and smaller. That's why you will take the biggest circumference and watch its changing. Also – you do not need to take the measures at one and the same place every time – taking the measures is quite subjective and not a stable parameter. You can monitor just one of the thighs – if the left is slimming, the right is also slimming for sure. It's just normal that there is a certain difference between the circumferences of the left and right thigh.

If you need to lose more than ten kilos then the scales might be of some help. Just don't use them every day but in larger periods like once a week. Then have in mind that the weigh will vary by a couple of kilos anyway. Measuring the weight is important when people have to lose much weight –

meaning for example women at about eighty kilos and height of 160 centimeters. In these cases monitoring the kilograms is helping and motivating.

But if you just need to improve your shape – get rid of the scale and buy a tape measure.

5 HOW TO QUIT THE SWEETS?

The most usual cause of the overweight is the sweet foods and the pastry.

If you are keeping a regime and you have gotten full with sweets and pastry – ok – what is done is done. But then you have to get back to your regime!

Let's face it – eating sweet things is like an addiction and the people who are addicted to sweet foods are probably more then the ones with some drug addiction.

You may not be quite conscious of that but you there is a serious battle in store for you here.

THE TASTE OF SWEET CAN CAUSE ADDICTION and if you are addicted you have long days of struggle in store for you. Abstinence is mental as well as physical. If your body is used to get quick calories by the sweets, it will want them again and again. You may have headaches for the first few days – from 3-4 up to 7 days in some cases. Usually it's after the seventh day you start controlling the want for sweet food but at that point if you have something sweet, even a small cram – it all starts again. But there are people who can get satisfaction by two pieces of chocolate and then relax ok.

How to quit sweet

Stage one.

You may put your regime for eating sweet like this – have something sweet on a certain day of the week. For example, it can be on Saturdays when your family is gathered together. Or it may be Fridays when your physical sessions can be longer and you get something sweet as a reward. At that stage while you have set a regime of eating sweets on certain days, sweet is not forbidden to you. If you feel that you need to have a sweet bite at different time – ok – have some. Usually the idea that there is nothing forbidden to you makes you stronger. This stage may take about six months.

Second stage

The second stage is very similar to the first one but the sweet food must be domestic. That makes you a bit slower in respect with time and effort and that way eating sweet will be a bit lessened. Duration is about six months again.

Third stage

It is like the second one but you have to start lessening the flower and the sugar in your home made pastry. You may replace them with fruit. Six months.

The fourth stage

Here the hunger for sweet is well under control and you must not feel want of sugar any more. You are happy that your home made pastry is healthier and you are able to eat them when you decide and with pleasure and not under the dictate of hunger for sweet. That takes six months too.

I don't like word "healthy" because it means nothing. It can just indicate that someone has started to pay attention to his or her health. People who generally take care of the food they eat do not divide their choices for food by healthy and non-healthy because good food is all healthy in general.

Fifth stage

 You can watch people eat sweets and that does not make you insane for sweet food. By that time you wonder if you have been looking so crazy before. You feel quite happy that you are free of that already. You have sweets only when there is an occasion or celebration. Six months.

Sixth stage

Your mind is free of the thought of sweet food and if you get to think of it again – it is in the way that it is not good for you and you do not need it. That idea is clear in your mind. It is similar to drinking water from a puddle on the street. Your food is clean, you plan it and you don't want things that are not good for you.

Controlling the sweet is mission possible!

Once a week or better once a month, if you are able to wait, you eat sweets – what you want as much as you want.

It would be very well if on that day you make a good hard physical training and longer than usual. And on the next day you may start with some easy aerobics before breakfast – longer than twenty minutes. Easy aerobics means even pace. Rope skipping, running or bike riding are options too. My personal experience with such nasty days is not amongst the pleasant ones but you try it for yourself and see.

If you are able to get all right with small amounts of food, you can have a bite or two of biscuits or some chocolate every day. This does not mean that I approve or encourage you to do so. It only means that I understand that people are different and may need diverse approaches to things. We are also on different stages of our personal development and that of course doesn't mean that some are advanced and some are retarded.

If you endure great stress, quitting sweets or cigarettes will add pressure.

May be that is not the right time for you to get to these things. You can just read, get informed, develop the right attitude and be ready to start reducing sweet some day when stress is overcome.

Trying once and failed must not cause you to give up fighting against sweet addiction. Go on trying. You will be s surprised to discover how much easier it gets by every next try.

Additional information:

A friend of mine shared with me that she has been brave and strong to keep her regime during some fests and then on the next evening she totally lost control. She got full with all foods she thought she needed. As a result she got a severe diarrhea, shaking of arms and legs too. The only asset is that now she has a very bad memory of the event so next time when she dreams of getting full with food she will remember the sickness it causes. This is how things turn in favor of the person who struggles with his or her uncontrollable appetite – bad memories of "delicious" things. And her body obviously knows what is good for it and got quick on getting rid of the extra food by the diarrhea.

If you are keeping a regime and it happens that you overeat some time – ok – things happen. But do not give up your regime – get back to it. You are human, not a robot. You don't have to blame yourself for human weaknesses.

You have to get aware of the fact that quitting sweet is a change in your way of life and not just a campaign that will be over soon. Some days you will win some days you will lose. But if you don't give up the winning days will be more than the losing days and that is what counts.

At the beginning it may seem that winning is impossible but in some time you will be wondering how you could think so.

Now then! We are motivated and informed how to stop the sweet.

Let's get to how to lose X kilos for Y days. Which regime is most suitable for me?

I REPEAT THAT BECAUSE IT IS CRUCIAL TO KNOW THAT IN THE SLIMMIMG PROCESS:

1. eating regime alone burns muscles along with the fats;

2. eating regime combined with physical training leads to burning fats and building some muscles;

3. physical exercises alone do not lead to losing weight.

1. You decide to lose some kilos by only a diet. Diet is a nutrition regime involving shortage of energy – meaning you get smaller amounts of energy by your food regime then the needs of your body. That causes your body to release its energy supplies to cover its needs. Body has two resources of energy to use in that case – the fats and the muscles. If you do not exercise then muscles are easier for the body to use than the fats. Conversion of

substantial amounts of fat into energy takes considerable amounts of oxygen. That is why jogging is so popular for those who want to slim. Jogging increases the influx of oxygen in the body and that enhances the conversion of the body fats into energy.

You on the other hand, do not exercise but only keep diet – no increasing of the oxygen in the body – so you hardly burn any fats. But your body is burning your muscles to supplement the energy it needs. The result is that you lose weight but it is actually losing very little fats and much more muscles. In some time you are slimmer and your circumferences are smaller but you do not look healthy and happy but puffy and with low tonus – what is the use then that you have slimmed.

2. Slimming with diet and physical exercises. That is the right way!

Again – your body has a deficit of energy and it goes to the fats and the muscles for supply. Then you use your muscles every day or regularly so the body "knows" that you need them every day so it keeps them fit (or takes some amount but little) and goes to the fats for energy. Your body is very clever and does not burn tissue that is so much needed. In addition your exercising is increasing the influx oxygen in the tissues and thus creates the proper environment for burning the fats and supplying you with energy.

3. Why not only exercises?

An hour of exercises burns 300-600 calories on the average depending on the intensity of the effort. Most of the people exercise very mildly though – no more then needed to just say they have carried out that task. You may be sure that your training is light by: feeling no want for breath, no panting and gasping, no pain in the muscles and not reaching the limits of the muscles (not all the time but it is needed from time to time), if after training you are not wet with sweat or you do not feel that your muscles are exhausted (in a good sense, of course); also - if you haven't been able to feel your pulse without touching your vanes…

In a nut shell – if you do not feel the difficulties of the exercising, you do not spend many calories and respectively your benefits of the quicker pace of metabolism after the sport session are very poor.

Say that you burn 200-300 calories in one sports session. In a glass of fresh fruit juice there are more calories than that. The same is true for a cup of coffee with sugar and cream plus a few biscuits. Then how do you intend to slim if the energy deficit is so small? Physical training by itself is quite insufficient to create energy deficit and to lead to slimming that way.

Then you decide to add food restrictions to your training regime. But food restrictions do not mean anything! You need a precise plan what to eat and how much, especially if you have tried to slim several times with no results. If you make the same mistakes every time the result will be all the same. Who has said that?

In other words – if you cannot slim by food restriction and a little more exercising – then obviously that is of no use to you and you need some thing that has proven to be effective.

The only way to make your belly flat and reduce your circumferences – hips, thighs, arms – this is a dietary regime that is able to create energy deficit combined with exercising the whole body (not only exercises for the belly, for example).

Now – let's get on the training sessions.

You have to understand how important they are and I promise that I'll help you to gain the best shape you have ever had no matter how old you are.

Training sessions

Exercises have a very important role.

They make the muscles fit and that improves your looks. The other important task of the exercises is to make the body burn fat and not muscles.

The main goal of slimming is to reduce the body fats and keep the muscles so that the body would be fit and good looking and sexy. Muscles are important to you if you want to look well after slimming (you certainly know that you have some muscles too – like the body builders but not so well in relief).

20 minutes of training are 1 % of your day time.

Are you still looking for excuses?

Most of the people succeed to reduce their weigh by training sessions once a day for about 12 minutes – for what matters is to exercise with leaving the zone of comfort for a while and not so much the duration.

You can train at home and you **do not really** need devices. You can use a mat or a blanket, a chair too. You can use only dumbbells for the back but if you don't have them you can use bottles of mineral water weighing 1.5 to 7 kilos (14 pounds).

A training session consists of warming, exercising and relaxing the muscles. These three parts take 40-45 minutes a day with the bigger effort at the exercising part that does not exceed 30 minutes. Every day you do different exercises so that you are not getting bored and exercise with pleasure.

Really, it's true that long walking, jogging or bike riding will do the same job. Yet if you want to refine your body you will have to do exercises. At the end of the book you will find links presenting exercises that you may use exactly as they are. They are there to help you.

These training models do not produce huge muscles. If you want to build muscles you will need the fitness saloons!

You are sure to slim though and not only this. You are gaining back your health – you will not need pills for the blood pressure, your cholesterol will get within the limits, your sleep will be improved, you will have more energy and you quality of life will be substantially improved.

HOW TO MAKE THE BELLY FLAT

One of the popular deceptions is that if you exercise a certain part of the body you can improve just that part preferentially. If people want to reduce their bellies they start training belly muscles – by crunches.

Or do exercises for the arms to reduce arm circumferences.

Both examples result by the same thing – the muscles trained are getting stronger. That does not mean that the fats there are burnt.

You have to look at your body as a whole organism and not as a gathering of parts. As you eat you supply energy for the whole body (and not for the different parts) and if you do not spend this energy it will be accumulated in the form of body fats.

For better visualizing the idea of that your body has a central source of energy imagine that while running you are spending the resources of that central energy store.

For better visualizing the idea of that your body has a central source of energy imagine that while running you are spending the resources of that central energy store.

Whatever exercise you do – all the same you are spending the reserves of that central store again.

So while exercising abdominal muscles you do not burn that fat there but you burn the energy stored in your body as a whole organism.

Accumulating of fats

When u receive more food, e.g. energy than you burn off you will have your body accumulating the spare energy as hypodermic fats. Different people accumulate fats in a different way. It means that if two different people eat more than their bodies' needs of calories they will accumulate the fats at different parts of their bodies. That is due to the different genes they have.

Men usually accumulate fats at their bellies and that is the popular beer belly and pouches even though many men with beer belly do not drink beer.

Women tend to accumulate fats on their thighs (mostly the inner and the rear part of them) and on the bottom.

These patterns of accumulating fat are connected with the hormones.

I give them for you, the reader to know that it is out of your hands to choose or manipulate the places where the fats will go once you have received more food than needed.

Burning of fats

When the body needs energy it addresses its reserves and starts burning them. If these reserves are stored at the belly – like men's bodies usually do, then the body will burn them. If it's a woman – the body will use the fats that have accumulated at the woman's thighs.

We usually burn the fats from where we have accumulated them. Meaning – if you want to put down your belly because it is too fat then most probably this will happen once you start eating less calories than you burn.

What are the most effective slimming exercises for big bellies?

It is obvious now that no matter which parts of the body you use for exercising you burn energy coming from the resources of your whole body. Then it is logical that the most effective slimming exercises are the ones that burn more energy and that are namely the biggest muscles of the body. These are:

- gluteus maximus or the bottom

- back

- thighs

- chest muscles.

It means that training your gluteus maximus/bottom, back, thighs or chest muscles you actually increase the speed at which you burn your body reserves (fats) and that of course will reduce the size of your belly or any part that your body tends to store its energy reserves. That means no matter where your body tends to accumulate the fats you have to train these four groups of muscles anyway.

That is why training styles that involve the whole body is the most effective way to burn off the fats not only at the tummy but all the fats of the body.

Another example is if you want to slim your arms you have to train the biggest muscle groups. When your training stows the back and the chest it also involves the biceps and the triceps and you can understand now that you actually burn far more energy that way than you might have burned training only the biceps and the triceps.

What should we do to reduce the tummy? It sounds funny to me to put the question that way – slim the tummy, the bottom, the arms – but this is the wording people use every day!

Most often when people want to slim they get to think about exercising for the sake of burning more energy. But in reality the role of the energy burning for the sake of slimming is far exaggerated. Here I do not speak of professional sports people.

In general one hour of training consumes about 300-500 calories but it is more likely that it would be rather 300 then 500. Here I speak of a training session at fitness saloons where you are usually offered exercises using no more than fifty percent of your muscles capacity.

Now – a piece of cake contains 300-400 calories.

A glass of fruit juice contains about 100 calories.

Small pack of biscuits contains about 300 calories.

That is easy to calculate – an hour at the gym will probably burn off the extra food you have eaten but not if it's more than 300 calories. And if it's more than that, you will be training and getting fat anyway. So obviously training cannot provide that deficit of calories that will make your body use the fats stored before and start the slimming process.

I have to tell you that- it's much easier NOT TO EAT these extra 300 calories than burn them by extra exercising. You better force yourself not to have these two glasses of juice or spare the packet of biscuits and you will not have to fight with these 500 extra calories. But if you want to burn 500 calories by exercising you will certainly have to get to heavy training for an hour or you will need several hours of milder exercising.

In short – sliming without diet based on calorie deficit is really DIFFICULT.

WHY train then – if it burns so little calories for me?

The role of the physical stowing is different then most people presume. Calorie deficit leads to two possible options for the body to cope with it – draw energy from the muscles or from the fats. If you only stick to dietary regime your body will use these two sources of energy. But if you exercise it is more likely that you would burn down only fats or fats mainly, not so much muscles.

I put here more likely because there are too many variants and people are too different but still in most of the cases when people exercise and keep a dietary regime along with it the result is that they burn mainly fats and not their muscles. It depends on the diet itself though but let us put here as granted that they get enough proteins and carbohydrates to make things simple.

Training increases the mass of the muscles and that is good for both men and women. And I mean it – for women too. Once they start training they usually build up muscles at the beginning but it does not go on for too long because of the lower levels of testosterone they produce. So it is hardly possible that they might put up too much muscle tissue.

Next, the body is using certain amount of energy so it is good that you have built up some more muscles so that you burn energy even in times when you do not use the muscles at all. Even if it's not too much energy consuming it adds to all the consumption so – step by step you can go far.

6 WHAT TO EAT

I offer that you should go through the dietary regimes I have prepared. As I have mentioned before, there is no popular dietary regime that I haven't studied and tried out. All these trials have brought me to a certain conclusion. If you want long term results you have to stick to high protein and law carbohydrate regimes and combine this nutrition with sport. That nutrition style is not too difficult to stick to and it can be very tasty too.

I offer several variants of a dietary regime with carbohydrates deficit.

That kind of regimes show results even in the first week. It depends on you if it would go on working for you later on too. I recommend that you do not give it up and go on for at least two weeks.

Once you have achieved the sliming result you have longed for, you should not go back to your past eating patterns or you will put on weight again. It does not mean you are entitled to stick to a diet for life. No way, I promise!

After slimming you better eat natural life foods like vegetables, fruit, meat, fish, cereals, pulses, cheeses, nuts. If that would be your choice of food you will not need to be careful with the quantities you eat and still you will be healthy and beautiful.

 So what to eat?

Protein diet - this is probably the most effective diet, especially when combined with exercise.

A Protein diet is to eat foods rich in protein,

Foods that are rich in protein:

● beef fillet, chicken, duck, whitefish and tuna.

- egg white

- non-fat yogurt (but carbohydrates in it have more protein)

- cottage cheese and non fat cheeses

- skim tofu

- all seafood

In general, there are a variety of foods rich in protein and low in fat and carbohydrates. Most foods in their natural state have the three major nutrients.

The main principle of any protein diet is to restrict intake of foods which are easily converted into fat, to eat mainly high protein diet in order to keep your muscles fit and combine this diet with exercise to keep your muscle mass.

I often dwell on the importance of only subcutaneous fats being removed, but not subcutaneous fats and muscles. The principle is simple: when there is a shortage of energy, the body begins to break down fat and muscle to provide energy.

To make the body "think" that the muscles can not be used for energy you need to make sure that the muscles are often used - i.e. if you do exercise your body, it will "think" that the muscles are necessary to sustain life and will only degrade fat.

Protein diet strongly supports this principle because protein is food for the muscles, it can be stored as body fat only if taken more than necessary.

It is customary for men's protein dose to be 3 grams (3.2 g) per kilogram of body weight, i.e. 80 kg man may accept 3 X 80 = 240 grams of protein a day.

Women's protein intake is less than 3 grams; think of 2.5 grams per kilogram of body weight, i.e. 60 kg woman can take 2.5 X 60 = 150 grams of protein a day.

What else can you eat while on the protein diet?

Fresh salad and vegetables are recommended. At least there are a lot of salads at any time of the year - tomatoes, cucumbers, lettuce, cabbage - can be eaten in unlimited quantities. Especially tomatoes contain lycopene, which is thought to increase the effect of protein diet (in truth one would need quite a lot tomatoes to eat as to feel the benefits of lycopene; tomatoes still are not a dietary supplement where the substances are concentrated in content). Popular in recent years French nutritionist Pierre Dukan, pronounced himself in favour of a few days /3, 5, 7 days/ deficit of vegetables in the diet in order to lose weight faster. I support his list of foods as the best source of protein food. I disagree with the lack of vegetables, which are a source of fibre. But overall a week without fibre is not something scary and definitely eating foods high in protein and low in carbohydrates will lead to the desired weight loss. His offer for a period with mixed foods (vegetables and protein) presents very well my understanding of protein diet; I think vegetables can be eaten every day and mostly raw to make the most of the vitamins and minerals in them. Thus you can distinguish right from wrong vegetables for protein diet, namely those that require cooking (beans, rice, potatoes, peas ...) contain carbohydrates and should be avoided.

What NOT to eat on protein diet

Sweets are banned - even fruits (though if you like to eat sweet then fruit is the better option). Forget about cakes, biscuits, pastries - if something tastes sweet - do not eat it. (Well, you will miss it, right? Remember how did we get here)?

Pasties - NO - this includes bread, pasta, and spaghetti.

Forbidden food processing is frying and breaded in particular.

Schedule meals at protein diet

It is better to eat 7-8 times a day, which is unrealistic for people who work. So I will explain the principle, and any reader can observe and adjust it according to their lifestyle.

The idea is to never go hungry and never be sated. If you keep on feeling too hungry the chance to break your diet is huge. Therefore you better eat every 2 hours.

Sample day when your protein diet

7-8 h a.m. - breakfast (a cup of skimmed yogurt)

10:00 h - breakfast (tomato salad with 150 grams curd and salt)

12:00 h - lunch (150 grams of meat on the grill and salad)

14 h- afternoon snack (a cup of skimmed yogurt)

16 h - late afternoon breakfast (egg whites with spices and salad)

18 h - Dinner (150 g grilled meat and salad)

20 h - light late dinner (soup with tofu)

There are thousands of variants for the preparation of tasty foods rich in proteins. You can be sate all day and your measures will be dramatically decreasing. I will advise you to trust your imagination if you need to make your own recipes. I can guess that it will be in several volumes.

PROTEIN DIET FOR VEGANS

It is very difficult to lose weight when you're a vegetarian, especially relying on protein diet because most protein sources are of animal origin.

The diet above is protein diet for people who eat meat.

Protein diet for vegetarians can be made for a period of 2-3-4 weeks and then you should start to eat richer variety of foods because eating the same diet for a long period of time is not healthy.

The concept here is to set a meal with proteins and combine them with good (poor and slow) carbohydrates (as no vegetarian foods only contain protein).

Best vegetarian protein source is the tofu. I know most of you do not like it, but that's because you never cook it properly. Lower in the diet has delicious recipes with tofu.

Monday - 1100 calories

Breakfast - 100 grams of raw avocado (160 calories) with tomatoes (eat them on the belly) and 50 grams low fat tofu (70 calories). Cut the avocados and the tomatoes; add a little salt and vinegar. Do not add olive oil because avocados are rich enough in oil. If you do not have avocado, then add 3 tablespoons of olive oil Extra virgin (not oil).

Snack - a medium-sized apple (200 grams). If you can - drink a dose of soy protein shake.

Lunch - 100 g cooked brown rice (110 calories) 150 g low-fat tofu (210 calories). You can boil the rice and tofu together with some spices - necessarily add much to taste (pepper, paprika, savory ...), do not put fat. Brown rice, if not pre- soaked needs half an hour boil! Salad - tomatoes and cucumbers or lettuce is also permitted.

After lunch you may have a glass of low fat soy milk. I personally did not like the taste, drink it through a straw so that it enters directly into the throat (sorry, but this package is protein diet for vegetarians). This is 80-100 calories depending on the brand of the soy milk.

Dinner - a bowl of lentil soup thick; about 200 g drained lentils. This is about 220 calories.

Tuesday - 1150 calories

Breakfast - a banana about 200 grams - 180 calories.

Snack - a glass of low fat milk or soy protein shake.

Lunch - boil 200 grams broccoli (70 calories) 200 grams low fat tofu (280 calories). Cut broccoli and tofu into small pieces, add salt and cook for 10 minutes, drain and eat.

Afternoon - 50 g raw walnuts - 320 calories.

Dinner - Boil a cup of peas with 2 chopped tomatoes, add spices. Serve with parsley. That comes to 200 calories.

Wednesday - 1400 calories

Breakfast - pour boiling water 3 tablespoons of oatmeal - 200 calories, add half a tablespoon of honey - 150 calories.

Snack - 50 g raw almonds - 280 calories.

Lunch - Cut zucchini 200 g (30 calories), add 200 grams of low fat tofu (280 calories), and bake in the oven for 20-30 minutes. Serve with dill.

Afternoon - a pear and a protein shake - 200 calories.

Dinner - a big bowl of bean stew, cooked without fat or a little olive oil (to account for no more than one tablespoon of olive oil per person or a cup).

Thursday - 1150 calories

Breakfast - 100 g of bread (about 2 slices Bonus) crush a raw tomato 50 grams low fat tofu, a little salt, rub the bread with the mixture.

Snack – a dose of protein shake.

Lunch - 200 g cooked potatoes with 100 g of tofu.

After lunch – have an apple.

Dinner - soup, tofu and leek. Cut 200 grams tofu, leeks and cook with garlic and salt for about 20 minutes.

I'm sorry if you are tired of tofu, but this is the best source of protein for vegetarians.

Friday - 1100 calories

Breakfast - 300 g kiwi

Snack - 50 g raw pumpkin seeds (unshelled).

Lunch - 200 grams of tofu, cook with two chopped tomatoes, add a tablespoon of olive oil and cook for 20 minutes. Serve with basil.

Afternoon - 200 grams of raw carrots. Wash and cut them lengthwise into thin strips. Squeeze a lemon into a cup, add salt and place the carrot strips in a bowl. Thus the carrots become more juicy and delicious.

Dinner - 300 grams of cooked lentils, you can cook with vegetables - tomatoes, carrots, garlic.

Saturday - 1100 calories

Breakfast – a large grapefruit

Snack - 200 g raw red peppers.

Lunch - 200 g spinach sauté with 200 g tofu, add a tablespoon of olive oil, salt and spices.

Afternoon - 50 grams of raw almonds.

Dinner - Stew 200 g potatoes 2 tomatoes, 2 red peppers and some garlic, add spices to taste.

Sunday - 1300 calories

Snack - an apple

Snack - 300 grams of melon (or still apples).

Lunch - 200 g spaghetti (200 g after being cooked). Prepare tomato sauce and tofu. Stew 100 grams tofu with 2 chopped tomatoes.

Afternoon - protein shake or 50 g raw hazelnuts.

Dinner - a bowl thick lentil soup - 300 grams.

Additional information on protein diet for vegetarians:

If 1100-1300 calories a day are too small for you, then add on another 2 fruits per day, one in the morning, the other for an afternoon snack. You can also increase the amount of tofu.

Protein diet shakes are not mandatory and is not usually recommended their frequent drinking, but since this is an easy way to obtain protein, so included. It's ok to drink protein shakes, problem is if you eat with them and eat a meal that needs strong digestion. Where to find a protein shake? In special shops for nutrition additives may be. Usually people who train in the gym know where the good stores are. What's suitable for vegetarians is soy protein but look that there is no sugar and carbohydrates - have them below 15%. Usually the package comes with a measuring spoon in. Take one dose, pour in a little water and whisk, then add a little more water - this is a protein shake.

Tofu, especially low-fat, is an excellent source of protein especially for vegetarians. There are different types / brands of tofu and they have a different taste. Try them out to find the one you like the most (some prefer tofu cooked in a soup or something but not clean).

Nuts are very healthy but high calories. For the period of the diet limit it to 50 grams per a meal.

Vegetables - eat them on the stomach - no restrictions because they contain fiber and help your body to throw out toxins and keep your belly full (decreases appetite). If in the evenings before falling asleep you feel hungry then have a salad as big as you want just do not put oil. Salt and vinegar are allowed in some reasonable amount and a tablespoon olive oil. Put limit on vegetables like potatoes because they contain a lot of carbohydrates.

If you are a vegetarian who eats milk, eggs and cheese, then you can replace tofu with egg whites. 100 g tofu can be replaced with 3-4 egg whites. Cheese you can eat up to 100 grams per day. Whites of the eggs are 100% protein, so for them there is no limit, but cheese is greasy, so put some restriction with it.

MORE FOR VEGAN / OR FASTING

If until now you did not know about the dangers in vegan food and still consume them safe and sound then you do not have to panic by what you will read now – I'd just like to inform you, not to scare and embarrass. I'm not telling you that if I do not follow these practices there is an immediate danger. Millions of people do not, including me; people do not always have the opportunity to observe everything by the rules.

So which foods to include in our fasts (or in case you're vegan) so you do not get fat?

Many people do not know that you can gain weight while eating super clean (no sugar, fried and processed foods). I.e. food below can cause increase of weight depending on intake levels.

We start with seeds

They contain many nutrients because their role is to keep the new generation and give a new life. Therefore they are supplied with defensive weapons to make anyone who eats them feel bad and the next time to pass or to eat less - so ensure the continuation of life. Seeds contain lecithin, toxins and phytates (phytic acid*) - it is their defensive weapons. Seeds put down their guard when there are favorable conditions to give life - say moist soil. To neutralize the weapons of seeds they should be soaked. If you have your breakfast seeds soaked in the night before then in the morning wash them and then eat.

Phytic acid* - this is the form in which the plants stored phosphorus; once in the digestive system they block the absorption of minerals - zinc , iron, magnesium and others.

Phytase is an enzyme that neutralizes phytic acid and has phosphorus released. This enzyme is found in plants which contain some phytic acid. In order to activate the enzyme phytase, the plants have to be soaked in an warm environment and then cooked. Some people have a greater ability to produce phytase by bacteria in the digestive system and therefore have a greater tolerance to foods that contain phytic acid.

Edible seeds - sesame, linseed, hemp, pumpkin seeds, chia.

Cooking, soaking and sprouting ** are the ways of disarming the seeds. Cook them at low temperature, slowly, to prevent possible oxidation of the fat therein. Oxidation of omega-3 fatty acids is reduced if during warming you add oregano or rosemary (rosemary is more efficient than oregano).

Whether the oregano would be as effective with the seeds we do not know, but it must not stop you from putting oregano while you roast nuts in the pan.

Nuts

Nuts also contain phytic acid. It is good practice to soak them for 18 hours and then dry it at low oven (about 50 degrees). If you eat a lot of nuts you can prepare 0.5-1 kg. Thus because preparing only 50 g of nuts seems uneconomical in terms of time and efforts having in mind the whole procedure.

Vegetables

In terms of energy, one can eat vegetables to the belly - raw, cooked, and roasted - and you can tolerate.

Fruits

Let the fruits be "the sweet food" in your menu.

Tip: Let the regime that you follow be good and comfortable for you, though not perfect. If you do 80% of things on the schedule, 20% can be anything you want. For example, it is more important to practice regularly, even shortly than to be the perfect time according to some theory – e.g. convenience is a priority here. I've read so many theories about when to train ... my truth is - regularly at convenient times. If you're not comfortable with the time to train, sooner or later you will stop practicing. So no matter what a perfect rule may be, it is important to be persistent in what you're doing - feeding, training...

Legumes, cereals and more.

In the book of Timothy Ferris '4 hour body' he says that if you add kelp while cooking beans and lentils that would eliminate or significantly reduces gas emissions. I have not tried and examined this detail in my research.

Legumes and cereals also contain phytic acid. Their perfect preparation involves soaking in a warm place and then cooking.

Sprouts **

It is not yet clear whether all foods can germinate and thus become better for consumption.

Sample Day Vegan regime

Breakfast: one piece of fruit, 50 g nuts. You can grind / cut the fruit, crush some nuts, add cinnamon /cocoa/, optional stevia leaf powder, stir to mix all smooth mush. You can add a few tablespoons of water to make it moist, homogeneous mixture.

Lunch: Stuffed peppers with beans. A 100 gr of old beans (300g when boiled, drained weight of a can possibly, check that there is no sugar added). Beans mixed with grated carrot and zucchini, add spices to taste (oregano, paprika, if you like garlic, chili). The peppers are filled with bean mixture, baked / cooked up. In the presentation, sprinkle with parsley and a tablespoon of fat (olive oil, flaxseed oil).

Dinner: Gazpacho with avocado and seeds. Mash the tomatoes as you want (when you use ready of a can you check the ingredients, see there is no sugar there), add sliced medium avocado cubes, crushed sesame seeds 20 grams, 20 grams of hemp seed. Optionally add to the cold soup carrots, zucchini, spinach and more raw vegetables.

Or: If you prefer cooked soups - just cut the above listed products, add seasoning to taste, bake in the oven or cook on a skillet. Upon presentation sprinkle with parsley and a tablespoon fat.

Good luck with the protein diet for vegans!

7 LOW CARBOHYDRATE DIET

This is another name for the protein diet. However, it has carbohydrates but slow (good) not to accumulate as fat and at places we least want it. Low carbohydrate diet is one of the effective ways to lose weight. The problem with most diets is that they are complex; they require cooking and eating in certain hours. This low carbohydrates diet is designed to help people who are super busy and want to lose weight without cooking and elaborate schemes to follow .

In the morning you can drink coffee or tea better without sugar if you can and if you cannot then only a small spoon.

Before lunch snack - drink a pot of yogurt (whisk so you can drink it).

For lunch, eat as much as you want fillet; you can have only fillet or sirloin and salad (salad is fresh vegetables). Do not eat bread.

For dinner eat as much as you want fillet possibly with just a salad again of fresh vegetables.

If two times a day one eats 150 g fillet - these are 300 grams per day. Surely a big man will eat more than an average height woman, so everyone should decide for yourself and determines how much to eat - no limit on quantity, but it is important to see how much per a day so as to consider what is necessary for one week of low carbohydrate diet.

Shopping list for the week:

1. Coffee or tea.

2. 7 pots of yogurts - it can be a variety of different brands .

3. 2-3 pounds of fillet meat (if you eat 300g a day 7 days - 2 kg and 100 g per a week). Take 7 different types, each packaged separately so you will know that you are taking a bag of food for the day and have it provided at the office. For example: 300 grams chicken , 300 grams of ham , turkey 300 g, 300 g pork, 300 g of any other kind so 7 different types to a variety throughout the week.

4. Vegetables - if you can make salads - tomatoes, cucumbers, cabbage, onion, parsley, lettuce.

Additional foods that are allowed during the low carbohydrate diet:
● Eggs (cooked).
● Cheeses in small quantities because of their fat.
● Bread in small amounts - a slice per day.
● Olives - 5-10 a day.
● Oatmeal - 2 table spoons per a day.
● All fresh vegetables.
● Baked fish.
● Peas, beans, lentils - 3 times a week for lunch, a cup to be boiled, no bread, plus a salad.

Prohibited food and drink while you're on a low carbohydrate diet
● White bread
● Soft drinks – they contain a lot of sugar and are a major problem for many people because one can seamlessly drink a litre Coca-Cola and be very hungry at the same time; yet it is stuffed with sugar. If you are the type who drinks a lot of pop drinks – if you only quit them, you will lose weight.
● Alcohol, even beer;
● Sweet things! If it tastes sweet – do not eat it, even fruit;
● Fried foods;
● Rice - 2-3 tablespoons of cooked rice is not a problem, for example as a side dish of fillets, but no more than that.
● Potatoes - 100 g boiled potatoes per a day are also ok, but no more. For example, instead of one slice of whole grain bread you can eat 100 grams of cooked potatoes (by no means fried) or 2-3 tablespoons of cooked rice.
● Fruits - contain many carbohydrates. It's okay to eat an apple 2-3 times per week or one orange and may be another piece of fruit, but generally all fruits are rich in carbohydrates and you have to avoid them throughout your low carbohydrate diet.
● Juices - without any clue, you get loaded with carbohydrates. In addition - juices contain sugar, sweeteners and preservatives. If you need to drink juices anyway, then let them be fresh, but you have to consider that a cup of juice is made from 2-3 pieces of fruit and these are a lot of carbohydrates.
● Sauces –they are very dangerous as they are really packed with fats.
● Pizzas, cakes, pastries, cakes, crackers – if some food is made of dough - you have carbohydrates there.

8 SUMMER WEIGHT LOSS DIETS

The difference with other diets is that it has less meat and more vegetables and fruits – at least a bit (because now I owe you a small compromise with fruits).

Day 1

Breakfast: 1 cup yoghurt 3.6% fat with a tablespoon oatmeal (not granola and plain oatmeal, do not add sugar or honey). You may have a cup of coffee or tea without sugar. Add a glass of water. About 280 calories

Lunch: 3 scrambled eggs with vegetables (mish mash), a large bowl of fat-free cold summer soup of fresh raw products – like the Bulgarian tarator for example. Add a glass of water. About 250-300 calories.

Afternoon: 200g of strawberries. Add a glass of water. About 64 calories.

Dinner: Grilled fish (about 300g) with a huge salad at your choice of vegetables (only fresh ones, please, except for potatoes and corn) flavored with vinegar, salt and a tablespoon of olive oil. Add a glass of water. About 300 calories.

Note: On a day with a training session can you drink protein shake after the physical. After the protein shake it is necessary to have a minimum of one hour or preferably 1.5-2 hours break and then you may eat. If you do not drink protein shakes after your workout, it is important to eat after it.

Day 2:

Breakfast: Oatmeal with cheese (optional 3 tablespoons). Add a glass of water. About 250 calories.

Lunch: 200 g of poultry (breast) grilled with salad at your choice (excluding potatoes and corn, seasoned with salt, vinegar, a tablespoon olive oil). . About 350 calories.

Afternoon: 200 gr. Of cherries. Add a glass of water. About 126 calories.

Dinner: Stuffed peppers with cheese and 1 cup of fresh vegs soup. Add a glass of water. About 200 calories.

Day 3

Breakfast: two full grain pancakes. Add a glass of water. About 350-400 calories - breakfast for champions!

Lunch: 300 g grilled fish (you know the requirements and the options by now about your choice of a fish dish) with salad of your choice. Add a glass of water. About 300 calories.

Afternoon: 25g of hazelnuts. Add a glass of water. About 160 calories. Courgettes with yoghurt and garlic (do not fry but bake them. Eat to the belly. Add a glass of water.

Day 4

Breakfast: Toasted sandwich on one slice of bread with 25g of cheese and 50g of ham. Add a cup of yogurt and a glass of water. About 220 calories.

Lunch: 300g of grilled fish with salad of your choice. Add a glass of water. About 300 calories.

Afternoon: 200g of strawberries. Add a glass of water. About 64 calories.

Dinner: Green beans with yogurt eat to the belly. Add a glass of water.

Day 5

Breakfast: ½ cup yoghurt 3.6% fat and 200 g strawberries. Add a glass of water. About 200 calories.

Lunch: Mish mash with 3 eggs, without any fat. Milk soup bowl (no fat). Add a glass of water. About 300 calories.

Afternoon: 25g of almonds. Add a glass of water. About 150 calories.

Dinner, Soup of salmon (or other fish) / recipe ... /. Eat to the belly. Add a glass of water.

Eat fruit one hour before the main meal. Not in any case immediately after it! Exclude bananas and grapes!

9 DIET FOR HIGH CHOLESTEROL

High cholesterol (LDL; cholesterol) leads to heart problems, so high cholesterol diet is a diet to keep avoiding heart diseases.

Bad cholesterol and most diseases are directly related to how we eat. If you pay attention to your diet (diet is a way of eating, not fasting) you will lower the bad cholesterol and thus may reduce the risk of atherosclerosis (a disease in which you have your arteries blocked), which causes heart attacks and other heart diseases.

If the process of blocking the arteries has already started, you can slow down its speed as you eat healthy. With minor changes in lifestyle (diet + movement) you can slow down the process of narrowing arteries and even stop it.

Eat well – I will never get tired repeating that!

Dietetic principles below will help you lower the total cholesterol in your body, as well as bad cholesterol, reduces blood pressure, blood sugar and weight (to lose weight).

7 Diet tips for high cholesterol and risk of heart disease

1. Eat more vegetables, fruits, whole grains and legumes. These foods contain fiber that reduces bad cholesterol LDL.

2. Selected fatty foods. From oily to oily there is a big difference. Unsaturated (good) fats from fish and vegetables are beneficial. ANIMAL (saturated) fats are not useful. In general - reduce fat intake. Limit the intake

of fat from butter, chocolate and sweets (often it is not clear what kind of fats are there), fatty meat. Obtaining your fats mainly of fish (omega 3, fatty acids, which are very important for the heart and reducing bad cholesterol) and olive oil (Extra Virgin). High doses of omega 3 fats lower cholesterol and reduce the risk of heart diseases.

3. Eat a variety of foods and in the right amount of protein ones. The main culprit of bad cholesterol and heart disease are the animal fats that are found in meat and most often in sausages (salami, sausages, etc.).

Selective the meats you eat. Do not eat the sausages; you do not know what they contain. Try to bake a sausage and you will see how much fat it will give away. This fat raises your cholesterol. Dairy products are also culprits of bad cholesterol. However, if you eat more than one cup of yogurt a day, consider that these be low-fat products. But if you occasionally eat yogurt, you better choose the whole fat ones because yogurt fats are negligible when not consumed frequently. Watch out for hidden fats in sweets. I know they do not look greasy but actually often contain margarine, and also are very sweet and rich in calories. Foods with a combination of protein foods - not greasy meat, fish and pulses (beans, lentils, chickpeas, peas) contain vegetable protein.

4. Restrict the intake of cholesterol. Cholesterol that we intake increases the level of cholesterol in the blood. This means that you should eat less saturated fat (animal, vegetable oil, margarine), which means fewer calories and losing weight.

5. Eat regularly. May not be less every 2-3 hours, but at least try to have 3 or 4 meals per day. Missing one meal usually leads to overeating. Regular meals keep your blood sugar and metabolism to be active round the clock.

6. Reduce salt intake. This will reduce the blood pressure.

7. Drink fluids. Body is made of water and needs it because it means the life for it. Water purifies us and gives energy. Drinking sodas and juices is very bad (containing too much sugar besides other problems there). Drink tea and water.

8. Enjoy the food. Find the healthy foods you love and do not eat food that you do not. When you enjoy your meal and keep positive attitude to food and even pleasure that makes you feel good and it is unlikely in such a frame of mind that you would eat too much.

And finally, eat right and be physically active! Laziness is bad for you.

10 HOW TO EAT AFTER WEIGHT LOSS

How to eat AFTER weight loss?

As you like, but if you exclude from your diet the sweets, baked and fried foods you can eat as much as you want. We said above - any pizza or chocolate cake will not hurt once a week. But then I must do resistance training or go walking at least 10 km to burn out the extra calories.

How to eat so that we would not get back all the lost kilograms and more?

The basic principle of weight gain is NOT: Eat as much as you spend. In other words, eat as many calories as you expend.

No need to stay on a diet to avoid gaining weight. Once you have lost weight, you can eat normally and not gain weight.

However:

If you indulge in much food that is not fresh or made of dough or fried - you will gain weight again.

The idea is to eat healthy 3-5 times a day without treading and try to apply what you have learned from your diet. No problem one day to overeat (you have been to visit Mom or it is Christmas), but the next day, make a day of discharge - eat salad and drink tea (water).

Try to balance your diet. Eat healthy most of the time, if occasionally „overuse", then do the day of discharge.

It is up to you to enjoy food without gaining weight.

The more simple food you eat, the better. What is simple food? That is food not too much processed and cooked in a complicated and fancy way.

If you love meat, do not cook with a complex sauce, or don't boil, bake, fry and finally put some sauce on it. Imagine people 200-300 years ago - how they prepared meat - most likely boiled or roasted. The simpler the better.

Why do you pour your salad with mayonnaise - use just salt, olive oil (oil) and vinegar.

Eat waffles, cakes and chips - but from time to time. It is best not to eat but hard to live with the limitations, right? If this is not your main meal, but just occasionally treating - no problem.

All in all – after been following a diet you should eat the same style but gradually increasing the quantity with an emphasis on raw and unprocessed foods.

To be effective with any diet and lose weight quicker – you have to fast and have training ... no you cannot go without physical. Prepare yourself a three-month training plan. This plan you can draw with any fitness trainer, you can find videos on you tube. You'll have to sweat in order to have any lasting results.

Nutritional supplements for weight loss - because I know you spent a lot of money by now, let me tell you of what has a real good effect;

"Celulit" is a unique formula that is conducive to the most efficient use of energy released from the digestion of food. It is particularly effective in the fat burning process. It suppresses appetite, creates a feeling of fullness, and prevents the accumulation of excess fat in the body.

Indications

In obesity, cellulite, overweight.

Not recommended for children under 6 years old, pregnant and nursing mothers.

Dosage

2 capsules a day, one hour before meals.

L-Carnitine is a classical lypotropic formula with proven effect on degradation of fat, particularly effective in combination with diet and exercises. Increases the energetic capacity and stamina during heavy physical exercises, promotes the rapid recovery of the body.

Indications

It is used to reduce the weight as a factor in melting excess fat, regulating metabolism and accelerating metabolite process. It is assigned as an adjunctive therapy in primary and secondary deficiency of Levocarnitine.

Dosage

The daily intake complies with the weight.

Fat burners

Fat burners are harmless products that unlike thermogenic products have no side effects and can be used safely. The effect of these drugs is not as strong as with the thermogenic products but they do deserve to be preferred as they cause no side effects. The main component of the phosphate burners is L carnitine, which transports fatty cells to the mitochondria where they are "burnt", i.e. used for energy. This happens even without an active exercising. Due to this property the most preferred time of intake of the fat burners is 2-3 hours before exercise. This gives you additional energy from burning your fat supplies while you exercise, and you will achieve an effective workout along with burning your fats. Besides you can receive fat burners before any physical work also. If you are taking higher doses, it is advisable to split them into several doses. Necessities might be different depending on the particular product.

Foods that enhance metabolism

It is believed that certain foods and herbs can help to enhance your metabolism, which in return becomes a machine for fat burning. Of course, exercise and proper nutrition are at the forefront, but if you can give one small additional push even if less effective at burning fat, why not then use some of these advantages.

Many of them, such as celery and grapefruit are not scientifically proven in this respect but still it is believed that they help in practice. Apple cider and vinegar are a favorite condiment for many recipes but they are also used for fat burning.

Vitamin C is known for its favorable effects, so include citrus fruits in your eating plan - lemons, oranges, grapefruit, and kiwi. Do not forget that tomatoes are a vegetable with the highest content of vitamin C.

Pectin, to be found in apples and other fruits, acts in the same way as lecithin - absorbs fats.

Soy nuts and soy products are generally quite controversial, but soy is a source of lecithin, which breaks down fats. It blocks the accumulation of fatty deposits in the cells.

Garlic

Yes, it gives a great flavor and taste to each dish. But there is another function. Neutralize the fats. It is also a diuretic.

Essential fatty acids

They control your weight. It's about omega fats (Udos) - flaxseed flour and flaxseeds, hemp, pumpkin seeds, sunflower seeds, evening primrose, olives, nuts, avocados and almonds. They are essential when trying to burn fat because fat removal is completely unhealthy. You can replace the bad fats with the good ones!

Natural diuretics

They can also help you in this endeavor. They remove excess water in your body that causes you to swell. Here comes the green tea.

Here are all the perfect complements to your diet so as to achieve maximum results.

So enough for now! I'm sure you know what to do from here on! It might be pleasant to sit chatting and gossiping but I think you already know enough and it's time for you to get your act together! If you are lazy you have a problem but I recommend you get out of the comfort zone, because comfort is a place where you've been, and obviously you're not happy with it!